PREDIABETES RECIPES

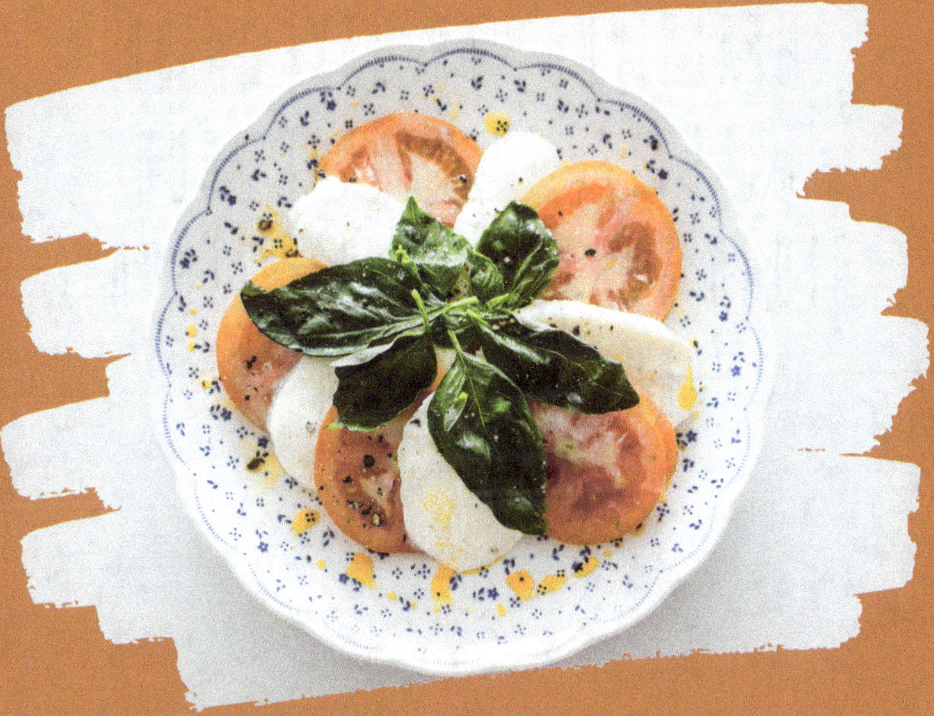

PEGGY R. MORGAN, RDN

PEGGY R. MORGAN, RDN

30 EASY & TASTY BALANCED MEALS YOU CAN MAKE IN 30 MINUTES, TO MANAGE YOUR BLOOD SUGAR LEVELS, WITHOUT SACRIFICING TASTE

ACKNOWLEDGMENT

I would like to express my heartfelt gratitude to everyone who contributed to the creation of "Prediabetes Recipes." This book would not have been possible without the support, encouragement, and expertise of the following individuals:

My family, for their unwavering encouragement and understanding during the writing process.

The dedicated team at I&O, whose guidance and expertise helped shape this book.

The healthcare professionals and nutrition experts who shared their valuable insights to ensure the accuracy and relevance of the recipes.

Friends and colleagues who provided inspiration and motivation throughout this journey.

The readers, whose interest in promoting health and well-being continues to drive my passion for creating nutritious and delicious recipes.

Thank you all for being a part of this project and for your invaluable contributions.

Peggy R. Morgan, RDN

ABOUT THE AUTHOR

Hey there, I'm Peggy R. Morgan, RDN – your culinary comrade, nutrition ninja, and the brains (and taste buds) behind these tasty creations! I'm on a mission to make your kitchen the coolest spot in the house, full of laughter, flavor, and downright deliciousness.

As a Registered Dietitian Nutritionist, I bring a blend of science-backed savvy and a whole lot of kitchen pizzazz to the mix. My love for all things food started in my grandma's kitchen, where I discovered the magic of fresh ingredients and the joy of sharing a meal with loved ones.

I'm not one to preach about the latest superfood trends. Instead, I'm all about a balanced and diverse approach to eating. Whether it's a hearty stew, a fresh salad, or a decadent dessert, I believe every meal should bring joy to your taste buds and nourishment to your body.

When I'm not playing mad scientist in the kitchen or doling out nutrition wisdom, catch me wandering local markets, sipping on herbal tea, or nose-deep in a good book. Because, let's face it, food isn't just about fuel; it's about feeding your spirit.

So, whether you're a kitchen pro or just figuring out where the spatula goes, join me on this flavorful adventure. Let's turn your kitchen into a place of endless possibilities, where every bite is a little celebration.

Stay tuned for more kitchen escapades as I whip up a storm in my upcoming books.

Connect with me (eatwithpeggymorgan@gmail.com) for updates and questions!

Ready to dive into the deliciousness? Let's cook up some magic together!

CONTENTS

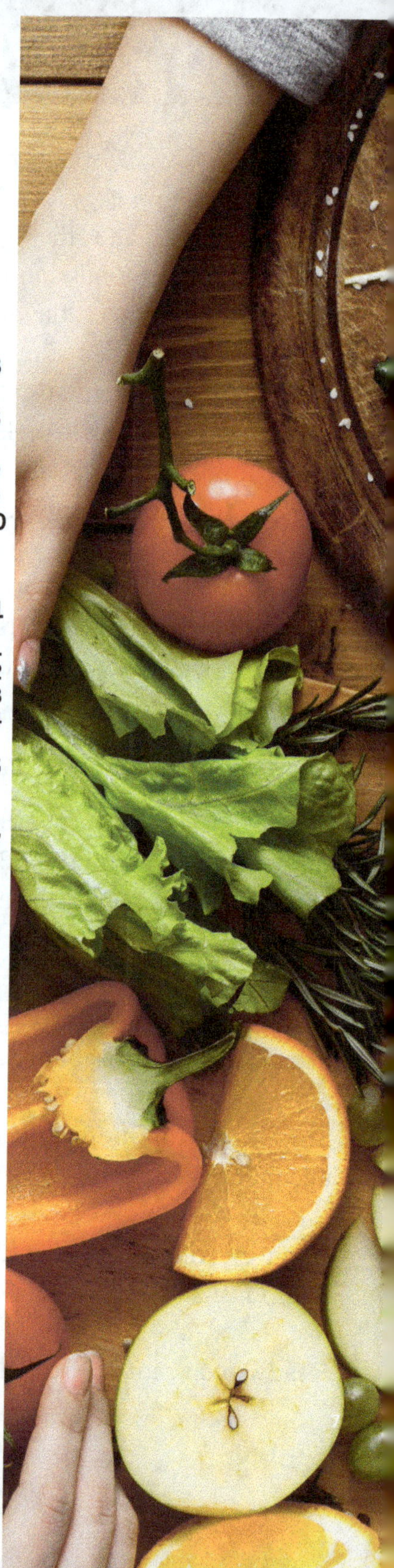

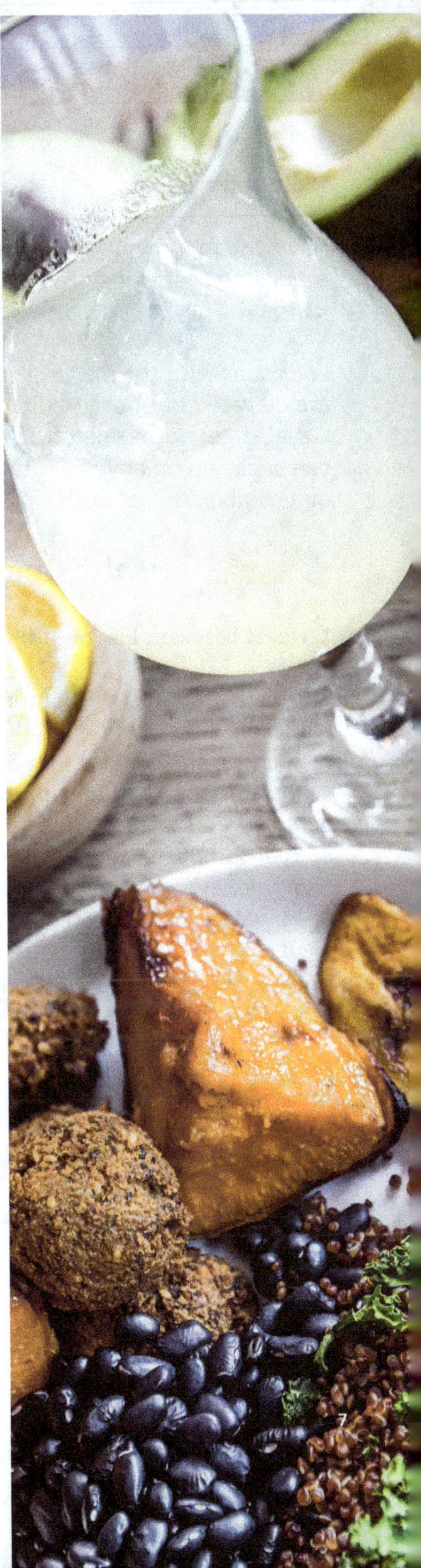

Hello and welcome,

Have you found yourself searching for a book that cuts straight to the heart of prediabetes, offering practical solutions and delicious recipes tailored for your journey? If so, you're in the right place.

Let's start with the basics: Prediabetes is a condition where blood sugar levels are elevated but not yet high enough to be classified as type 2 diabetes. It's a signal, a gentle warning from your body that a change is needed. Prediabetes can sneak up on anyone – it might be influenced by genetics, lifestyle choices, or a combination of both.

Health Complications of Prediabetes

1. Heart Disease: Elevated blood sugar levels can contribute to cardiovascular issues.
2. Type 2 Diabetes: Without intervention, prediabetes often progresses to full-blown diabetes.
3. Kidney Damage: Prolonged high blood sugar can impact kidney function.
4. Nerve Damage (Neuropathy): Uncontrolled blood sugar can lead to nerve damage, affecting sensation and function.
5. Eye Complications: Prediabetes increases the risk of diabetic retinopathy and other eye issues.
6. Increased Risk of Stroke: High blood sugar levels are associated with an elevated risk of stroke.

Essential Aspects of Managing Prediabetes

But, the good news is that it's a condition that can often be managed and even reversed through thoughtful choices. Beyond your diet, let's touch on other essential aspects of managing prediabetes. They include:

1. Healthy Eating: Embrace a balanced diet rich in fruits, vegetables, whole grains, lean proteins, and healthy fats.
2. Regular Exercise: Engage in physical activity to improve insulin sensitivity and support overall health.
3. Weight Management: Achieve and maintain a healthy weight to reduce the strain on your body.
4. Blood Sugar Monitoring: Keep track of your blood sugar levels regularly.
5. Stress Management: Practice stress-reducing activities like meditation or yoga.
6. Hydration: Drink plenty of water to aid digestion and overall well-being.

Key Terms

I won't drown you in medical jargon, but here are a few key terms to get us started.

1. Blood Glucose: The sugar in your blood, which comes from the food you eat and is a primary energy source for the body.
2. Insulin Resistance: When cells don't respond effectively to insulin, leading to elevated blood sugar levels.
3. Glycemic Index (GI): A measure of how quickly a food raises blood sugar levels.

And now, a promise: This book won't waste your time with unnecessary details. We're diving straight into the heart of it – the recipes. No lengthy monologues, just practical and delicious solutions to help you embrace a prediabetes-friendly lifestyle.

Remember, these lifestyle changes are not just a temporary fix but a sustainable approach to managing and even reversing prediabetes. Each small, positive choice adds up, contributing to a healthier and more vibrant life.

This book is designed to be your friendly companion on this journey, offering support and encouragement along the way. So, get ready to embark on a flavorful adventure that prioritizes your health. Let's turn the page and begin this journey together, one recipe at a time.

Foods to Avoid for Prediabetes

1. Added Sugars:
- Sodas, sugary beverages
- Candy, pastries, and desserts with added sugars
- Sweetened cereals and snacks

2. Refined Carbohydrates:
- White bread, white rice, and pasta
- Processed snacks and baked goods
- Sugary breakfast cereals

3. Highly Processed Foods:
- Fast food and fried items
- Processed meats (sausages, hot dogs)
- Packaged convenience meals

4. Saturated and Trans Fats:
- Deep-fried foods
- Processed meats
- Commercially baked goods

5. Excessive Salt:
- Highly salted snacks
- Processed and canned foods with added salt
- High-sodium condiments

6. Alcohol in Excess:
* Excessive consumption of alcoholic beverages

Foods to Embrace for Prediabetes

1. High-Fiber Foods:
* Whole grains (brown rice, quinoa, oats)
* Legumes (beans, lentils)
* Fruits (Berries, Apples, Citrus fruits) and non-starchy vegetables

2. Proteins (Lean):
* Skinless poultry
* Fish (especially fatty fish like salmon)
* Plant-based proteins (tofu, tempeh)
* Lean cuts of beef or pork
* Eggs in moderation

3. Healthy Fats:
* Avocados
* Nuts and seeds
* Olive oil

4. Colorful Vegetables:
* Leafy greens
* Cruciferous vegetables (broccoli, cauliflower)
* Colorful bell peppers, tomatoes, and carrots

5. Low-Fat Dairy or Dairy Alternatives:
* Greek yogurt
* Low-fat or fat-free milk
* Unsweetened almond or soy milk

6. Herbs and Spices:
* Fresh herbs (cilantro, basil)
* Spices (cinnamon, turmeric) for flavor without added calories

7. Hydration:
* Water
* Herbal teas

Remember, a balanced approach is key. Aim for variety in your diet, focusing on whole, nutrient-dense foods while being mindful of portion sizes. It's about creating sustainable habits that contribute to overall health and support your prediabetes management journey.

Always consult with healthcare professionals for personalized advice based on your specific health needs.

RECIPES

Egg and Veggie Muffins

SERVINGS : 2 | **PREP TIME** : 15 MIN | **COOKING TIME : 20 MIN**

RATINGS : 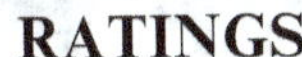 ★★★★★

INGREDIENTS

- 4 large eggs
- 1/4 cup (60 ml) unsweetened almond milk
- 1 cup (150 g) diced bell peppers (assorted colors)
- 1 cup (150 g) chopped spinach
- 1/2 cup (75 g) cherry tomatoes, halved
- 1/4 cup (30 g) diced red onion
- 2 tbsps. (30 ml) olive oil
- Salt and pepper to taste
- Cooking spray for greasing the muffin tin

METHOD

1. Preheat the oven to 350°F (175°C) and lightly grease a muffin tin with cooking spray.
2. In a skillet, heat olive oil over medium heat. Add diced bell peppers, chopped spinach, cherry tomatoes, and red onion. Sauté until the vegetables are tender, about 5 minutes. Set aside to cool.
3. In a mixing bowl, whisk together eggs and almond milk. Season with salt and pepper.
4. Distribute the sautéed vegetables evenly among the muffin tin cups.
5. Pour the egg mixture over the vegetables in each cup, filling about 2/3 full.
6. Bake in the preheated oven for approximately 15-20 minutes or until the eggs arc set.
7. Allow the muffins to cool for a few minutes before removing them from the tin.

Savory Cottage Cheese Pancakes

SERVINGS : 2   **PREP TIME** : 10 MIN   **COOKING TIME : 10 MIN**

RATINGS : 

INGREDIENTS

- 1 cup (240 ml) low-fat cottage cheese
- 2 large eggs
- 1/4 cup (30 g) almond flour
- 1/4 cup (30 g) coconut flour
- 1/4 cup (60 ml) unsweetened almond milk
- 1/4 cup (30 g) finely chopped chives
- Salt and pepper to taste
- 2 tablespoons (30 ml) olive oil for cooking

METHOD

1. In a mixing bowl, combine cottage cheese, eggs, almond flour, coconut flour, almond milk, chopped chives, salt, and pepper. Mix until well combined.
2. Heat olive oil in a non-stick skillet over medium heat.
3. Spoon the pancake batter onto the skillet, forming small pancakes. Cook for 3-4 minutes on each side or until golden brown.
4. Once cooked, transfer the pancakes to a plate.

Nutritional Value (Per Serving): Calories: 300 kcal, Carbohydrates: 15 g, Proteins: 25 g, Fats: 16 g, Sugar: 3 g

Mango and Mint Quinoa Porridge

🍴 SERVINGS : 2   🕐 PREP TIME : 10 MIN   🕐 COOKING TIME : 15 MIN

RATINGS :  ★★★★★

INGREDIENTS

- 1 cup quinoa, rinsed (185g)
- 2 cups water (475ml)
- 1 ripe mango, diced (200g)
- Fresh mint leaves, finely chopped (2 tbsps.)
- 1/4 cup unsweetened almond milk (60ml)
- 2 tbsps. chopped almonds (30g)
- 1 tbsp. chia seeds (15g)
- 1/2 tsp vanilla extract
- Pinch of salt

METHOD

1. In a saucepan, combine rinsed quinoa and water. Bring to a boil, then reduce heat, cover, and simmer for 15 minutes or until quinoa is cooked and water is absorbed.
2. Once cooked, fluff the quinoa with a fork and let it cool slightly.
3. In a mixing bowl, combine the cooked quinoa, diced mango, chopped mint, almond milk, chopped almonds, chia seeds, vanilla extract, and a pinch of salt. Mix well.
4. Divide the mixture into two serving bowls.
5. Top each bowl with additional mango slices, mint leaves, and a sprinkle of chopped almonds

Nutritional Value (Per Serving): Calories: 320, Carbohydrates: 55g, Proteins: 9g, Fats: 7g, , Sugar: 17g.

Sweet Potato and Black Bean Breakfast Tacos

🍴 **SERVINGS : 2**   🕐 **PREP TIME** : 15 MIN   🕐 **COOKING TIME : 15 MIN**

RATINGS : ★★★★★

INGREDIENTS

- 1 medium-sized sweet potato, peeled and diced (about 200g or 1 cup)
- 1 cup canned black beans, drained and rinsed (about 240g)
- 4 large eggs
- 4 small corn tortillas
- 1 tablespoon olive oil (15ml)
- 1/2 teaspoon ground cumin
- 1/2 teaspoon smoked paprika
- Salt and pepper to taste
- Fresh cilantro, chopped, for garnish
- Salsa (sugar-free) for serving

METHOD

1. Heat olive oil in a skillet over medium heat.
2. Add diced sweet potatoes and cook until they start to soften, about 8-10 minutes.
3. Stir in cumin, smoked paprika, salt, and pepper.
4. Add black beans to the skillet and cook for an additional 3-5 minutes until heated through.
5. Push the sweet potato and black bean mixture to one side of the skillet, crack the eggs into the other side, and scramble until cooked.
6. Warm the corn tortillas in a dry pan or microwave.
7. Divide the sweet potato, black bean, and egg mixture among the tortillas.
8. Garnish with fresh cilantro and serve with salsa.

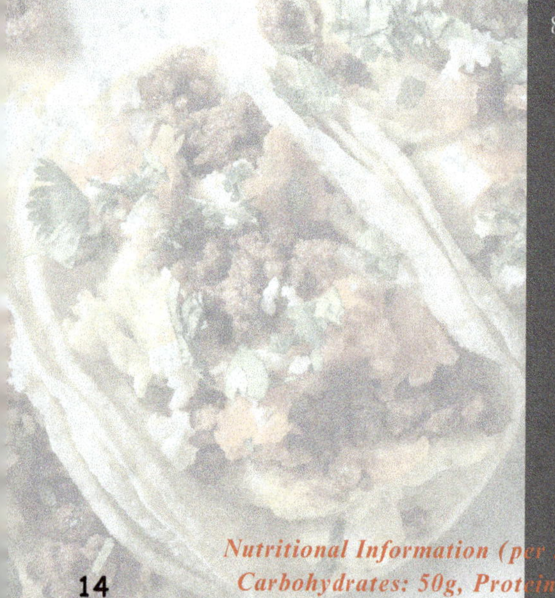

Nutritional Information (per serving): Calories: 400 kcal, Carbohydrates: 50g, Proteins: 18g, Fats: 15g, Sugar: 4g

Cranberry Walnut Baked Oatmeal Cups

SERVINGS : 2   **PREP TIME : 10 MIN**   **COOKING TIME : 20 MIN**

RATINGS : ★★★★★

INGREDIENTS

- 1 cup rolled oats (80g)
- 1/4 cup chopped walnuts (30g)
- 1/4 cup dried cranberries (40g)
- 1/2 teaspoon ground cinnamon
- 1/2 teaspoon baking powder
- 1/8 teaspoon salt
- 1 cup unsweetened almond milk (240ml)
- 1 large egg
- 1/2 teaspoon vanilla extract

METHOD

1. Preheat your oven to 350°F (180°C). Grease a muffin tin or line it with paper cups.
2. In a mixing bowl, combine the rolled oats, chopped walnuts, dried cranberries, ground cinnamon, baking powder, and salt.
3. In a separate bowl, whisk together the almond milk, egg, and vanilla extract.
4. Pour the wet ingredients into the dry ingredients and mix until well combined.
5. Divide the mixture evenly into the muffin cups.
6. Bake in the preheated oven for approximately 20 minutes or until the tops are golden brown and a toothpick comes out clean.
7. Allow the oatmeal cups to cool slightly before removing them from the muffin tin.

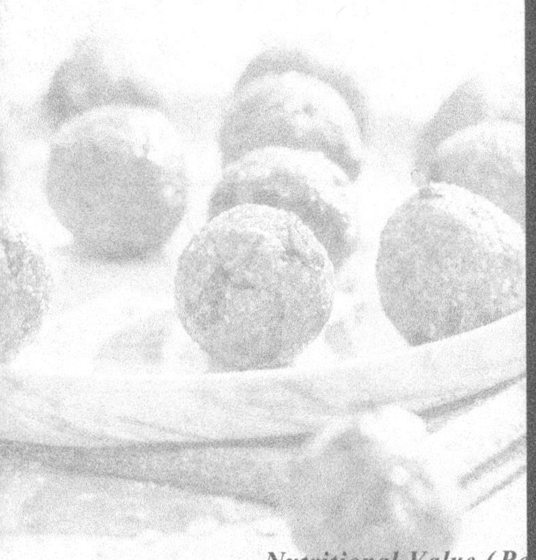

DAILY MEAL PLANNER

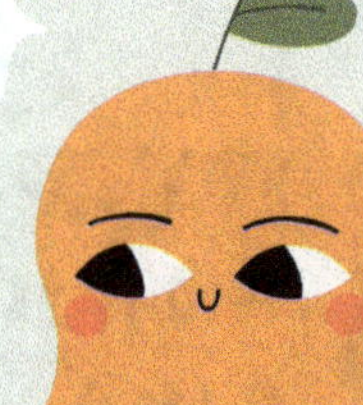

DAY/DATE: _______________________________

BREAKFAST

LUNCH

DINNER

SNACKS

GROCERY LIST

NOTES

____

____

____

____

Spicy Shrimp and Avocado Cabbage Wraps

SERVINGS : 2   **PREP TIME** : 15 MIN   **COOKING TIME : 10 MIN**

RATINGS :  ★★★★★

INGREDIENTS

- 200g shrimp, peeled and deveined
- 1 medium avocado, diced
- 2 cups shredded green cabbage
- 1/2 cup cherry tomatoes, halved
- 1/4 cup diced red onion
- 2 tablespoons chopped fresh cilantro
- 1 tablespoon olive oil
- 1 clove garlic, minced
- 1/2 teaspoon smoked paprika
- 1/4 teaspoon cayenne pepper (adjust to taste)
- Salt and pepper to taste
- 2 large cabbage leaves (for wrapping)

METHOD

1. In a medium bowl, toss the shrimp with olive oil, minced garlic, smoked paprika, cayenne pepper, salt, and pepper.
2. Heat a non-stick skillet over medium heat. Add the seasoned shrimp and cook for 2-3 minutes per side until they turn pink and opaque. Remove from heat.
3. In a large mixing bowl, combine shredded cabbage, diced avocado, cherry tomatoes, diced red onion, and chopped cilantro.
4. Add the cooked shrimp to the vegetable mixture and gently toss until well combined.
5. Place a portion of the shrimp and vegetable mixture onto each cabbage leaf, creating wraps.
6. Serve immediately, and enjoy these spicy shrimp and avocado cabbage wraps.

Nutritional Value (per serving): Calories: 280 kcal, Carbohydrates: 15g, Proteins: 20g, Fats: 18g, Sugar: 3g

Lemon Herb Tofu Skewers

SERVINGS : 2   **PREP TIME : 15 MIN**   **COOKING TIME : 15 MIN**

RATINGS : 

INGREDIENTS

- 200g extra-firm tofu, pressed and cubed
- 1 lemon, juiced and zested
- 2 tbsps. Olive oil
- 1 tsp dried oregano
- 1 tsp dried thyme
- 1 tsp garlic powder
- Salt and pepper to taste
- 1 zucchini, sliced into rounds
- 1 bell pepper, cut into chunks
- 1 cup cherry tomatoes
- Wooden skewers, soaked in water

METHOD

1. In a bowl, mix lemon juice, lemon zest, olive oil, oregano, thyme, garlic powder, salt, and pepper to create the marinade.
2. Cut tofu into bite-sized cubes and marinate for at least 10 minutes.
3. Preheat the grill or grill pan on medium heat.
4. Thread marinated tofu, zucchini rounds, bell pepper chunks, and cherry tomatoes onto the skewers.
5. Grill skewers for about 6-8 minutes, turning occasionally until tofu is golden and vegetables are tender.
6. Serve immediately.

Nutritional Value (per serving): Calories: 250, Carbohydrates: 15g, Proteins: 12g, Fats: 18g, Sugar: 5g

Sweet Potato and Black Bean Quesadillas

RATINGS : 

INGREDIENTS

- 1 medium sweet potato, peeled and grated (about 200g)
- 1 can (15 oz.) black beans, drained and rinsed
- 1 cup diced bell peppers (mix of colors)
- 1 cup chopped spinach
- 1 teaspoon ground cumin
- 1 teaspoon chili powder
- Salt and pepper to taste
- 4 whole wheat tortillas (8 inches each)
- 1 cup shredded lean cheese (cheddar, Monterey Jack, or a blend)

METHOD

1. In a bowl, mix grated sweet potato, black beans, diced bell peppers, chopped spinach, ground cumin, chili powder, salt, and pepper.
2. Heat a non-stick skillet over medium heat. Place one tortilla in the skillet.
3. Spread a quarter of the sweet potato and black bean mixture evenly over half of the tortilla.
4. Sprinkle a quarter of the shredded cheese over the mixture.
5. Fold the other half of the tortilla over the filling, creating a half-moon shape. Press down gently with a spatula.
6. Cook for 3-4 minutes on each side or until the tortilla is golden brown and the cheese is melted.
7. Repeat the process with the remaining tortillas and filling.
8. Once cooked, transfer the quesadillas to a cutting board and let them rest for a minute before slicing into wedges.

Sesame Ginger Turkey Lettuce Wraps

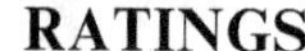 SERVINGS : 2 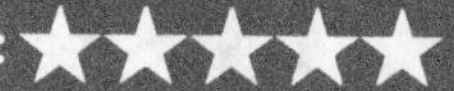 PREP TIME : 15 MIN   COOKING TIME : 10 MIN

RATINGS : ★★★★★

INGREDIENTS

- 250g (8.8 oz.) lean ground turkey
- 1 tablespoon sesame oil
- 2 tablespoons low-sodium soy sauce
- 1 tablespoon rice vinegar
- 1 teaspoon fresh ginger, grated
- 2 cloves garlic, minced
- 1 cup shredded cabbage
- 1 medium carrot, julienned
- 4 green onions, thinly sliced
- 1 tablespoon sesame seeds
- 1 head iceberg or butter lettuce, separated into leaves

METHOD

1. In a large skillet over medium heat, add sesame oil and brown the ground turkey until fully cooked.
2. Stir in soy sauce, rice vinegar, grated ginger, and minced garlic. Cook for an additional 2 minutes, allowing the flavors to meld.
3. Add shredded cabbage, julienned carrot, and sliced green onions. Cook for another 3-5 minutes until the vegetables are slightly tender.
4. Sprinkle sesame seeds over the mixture, stir well, and cook for an additional 1-2 minutes.
5. Carefully spoon the turkey mixture into individual lettuce leaves, creating wraps.
6. Serve immediately, and enjoy your Sesame Ginger Turkey Lettuce Wraps!

Nutritional Value (Per serving: Calories 230,
Carbohydrates: 12g, Prot...

Mushroom and Spinach Stuffed Chicken Breast

SERVINGS : 2   **PREP TIME : 15 MIN**   **COOKING TIME : 25 MIN**

RATINGS : 

INGREDIENTS

- 1 cup fresh spinach, chopped (30g)
- 1 cup mushrooms, finely chopped (100g)
- 2 cloves garlic, minced
- 1 tablespoon olive oil (15ml)
- 1 teaspoon dried thyme
- 1 teaspoon smoked paprika
- Salt and pepper to taste

METHOD

1. Preheat the oven to 375°F (190°C).
2. In a pan, heat olive oil over medium heat. Add garlic and sauté until fragrant.
3. Add chopped mushrooms to the pan and cook until they release their moisture and become golden brown. Stir in the chopped spinach and cook until wilted. Season with salt, pepper, dried thyme, and smoked paprika. Set aside to cool.
4. Butterfly each chicken breast by slicing horizontally, creating a pocket for the stuffing.
5. Stuff each chicken breast with the mushroom and spinach mixture, pressing down to secure the filling.
6. Season the outside of the chicken breasts with salt and pepper.
7. In an oven-safe skillet, heat olive oil over medium-high heat. Add stuffed chicken breasts and sear on each side until golden brown.
8. Transfer the skillet to the preheated oven and bake for 20 minutes or until the chicken reaches an internal temperature of 165°F (74°C).
9. Once cooked, remove from the oven and let it rest for a few minutes before slicing.

Nutritional Value (Per Serving): Calories: 250,
Carbohydrates: 5g, Protein: 31g, Fat: 10g, Sugar: 2g

DAILY MEAL PLANNER

DAY/DATE: ________________________

BREAKFAST

GROCERY LIST

LUNCH

DINNER

SNACKS

NOTES

Miso-Glazed Salmon with Bok Choy

SERVINGS : 2   **PREP TIME** : 10 MIN   **COOKING TIME : 15 MIN**

RATINGS : ★★★★★

INGREDIENTS

- 2 salmon fillets (approx. 6 oz. / 170 g each)
- 2 bok choy heads, halved
- 2 tablespoons white miso paste
- 1 tablespoon low-sodium soy sauce
- 1 tablespoon mirin
- 1 tablespoon rice vinegar
- 1 tablespoon grated fresh ginger
- 1 clove garlic, minced
- 1 teaspoon sesame oil
- Sesame seeds for garnish (optional)

METHOD

1. Preheat the oven to 400°F (200°C).
2. In a small bowl, mix miso paste, soy sauce, mirin, rice vinegar, grated ginger, and minced garlic to create the glaze.
3. Place salmon fillets on a lined baking sheet and brush the miso glaze generously over each fillet.
4. Arrange bok choy around the salmon, drizzle with sesame oil, and season with salt and pepper.
5. Bake in the preheated oven for 12-15 minutes or until salmon is cooked through and flakes easily.
6. Optional: Sprinkle sesame seeds over the salmon and bok choy before serving.

Nutritional Value (Per Serving): Calories: 380, Carbohydrates: 12g, Proteins: 38g, Fats: 20g, Sugar: 4g

Spaghetti Squash Primavera

🍴 **SERVINGS : 2**　　🕐 **PREP TIME** : 15 MIN　　🕐 **COOKING TIME : 20 MIN**

RATINGS : ★★★★★

INGREDIENTS

- 1 medium-sized spaghetti squash (Approximately 1 kg or 2.2 lbs.)
- 2 tbsps. Olive oil (30 ml)
- 1 cup cherry tomatoes, halved (150 g)
- 1 medium zucchini, julienned (200 g)
- 1 bell pepper (any color), thinly sliced (150 g)
- 2 cloves garlic, minced
- 200g lean chicken breast, cooked and shredded (7 oz.)
- 1 tsp Italian seasoning
- Salt and pepper to taste
- Fresh basil leaves for garnish

METHOD

1. Preheat the oven to 375°F (190°C).
2. Cut the spaghetti squash in half lengthwise. Scoop out the seeds and membranes. Place the halves on a baking sheet, cut side up.
3. Drizzle each half with 1 tablespoon of olive oil, and season with salt and pepper. Roast in the preheated oven for about 30 minutes or until the squash is tender.
4. In a large skillet, heat the remaining tablespoon of olive oil over medium heat. Add garlic, cherry tomatoes, zucchini, and bell pepper. Sauté until vegetables are tender-crisp.
5. Use a fork to scrape the spaghetti squash strands into the skillet. Add shredded chicken and Italian seasoning. Toss until well combined and heated through.
6. Season with salt and pepper to taste. Garnish with fresh basil leaves.
7. Divide the Spaghetti Squash Primavera into two servings and serve immediately.

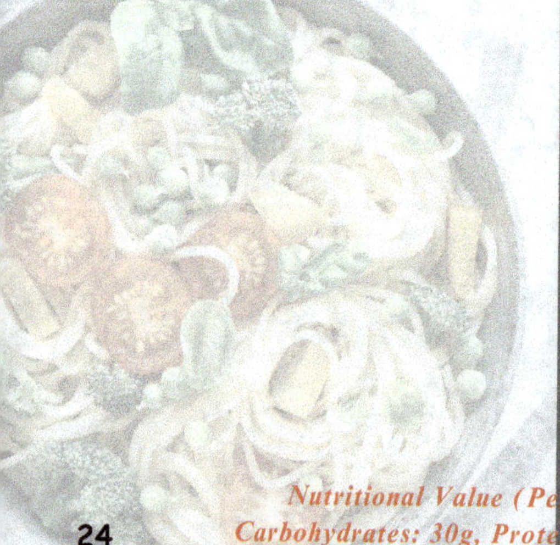

Nutritional Value (Per Serving): Calories: 320, Carbohydrates: 30g, Proteins: 25g, Fats: 12g, Sugar: 12g

Lemon Dill Baked Cod with Cabbage Slaw

🍴 **SERVINGS : 2**   🕐 **PREP TIME : 15 MIN**   🕐 **COOKING TIME : 15 MIN**

RATINGS : ★★★★★

INGREDIENTS

- 2 cod fillets (about 6 oz. each)
- 1 lemon (juiced and zested)
- 2 tablespoons olive oil
- 1 tablespoon fresh dill (chopped)
- Salt and pepper to taste
- Cabbage Slaw:
- 2 cups shredded cabbage
- 1/2 cup shredded carrots
- 2 tablespoons apple cider vinegar
- 1 tablespoon Dijon mustard
- 1 tablespoon olive oil
- Salt and pepper to taste

METHOD

1. Preheat the oven to 400°F (200°C).
2. In a small bowl, mix together lemon juice, lemon zest, olive oil, chopped dill, salt, and pepper to create the marinade.
3. Place the cod fillets in a baking dish and pour the marinade over them. Ensure the fillets are well coated. Let it marinate for 10 minutes.
4. While the cod is marinating, prepare the cabbage slaw. In a large bowl, combine shredded cabbage and carrots. In a separate small bowl, whisk together apple cider vinegar, Dijon mustard, olive oil, salt, and pepper. Pour the dressing over the cabbage mixture and toss until well combined.
5. Place the marinated cod in the preheated oven and bake for approximately 12-15 minutes or until the fish flakes easily with a fork.
6. Serve the lemon dill baked cod over a bed of cabbage slaw.

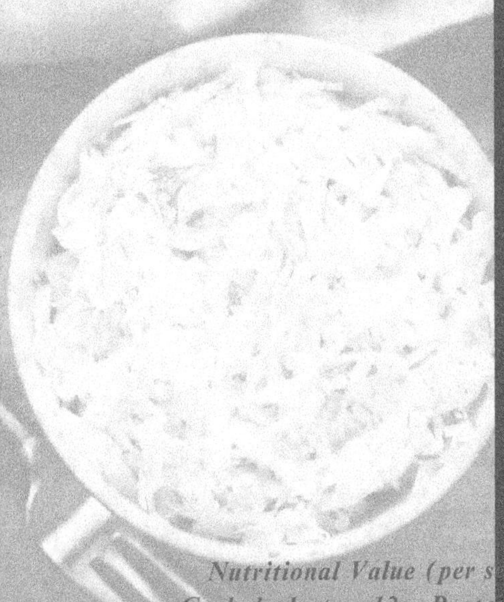

Asparagus and Goat Cheese Frittata

SERVINGS : 2   **PREP TIME : 10 MIN**   **COOKING TIME : 20 MIN**

RATINGS : 

INGREDIENTS

- 150g (5.3 oz.) fresh asparagus, trimmed and chopped
- 4 large eggs
- 60g (2 oz.) goat cheese, crumbled
- 1/4 cup (60ml) unsweetened almond milk
- 1 tbsp. (15ml) olive oil
- 1/4 tsp black pepper
- 1/4 tsp sea salt
- 1/2 tsp dried thyme

METHOD

1. Preheat the oven to 180°C (350°F).
2. In a medium bowl, whisk together eggs, almond milk, salt, pepper, and dried thyme.
3. Heat olive oil in an oven-safe skillet over medium heat. Add chopped asparagus and sauté for 3-4 minutes until slightly tender.
4. Pour the egg mixture over the asparagus in the skillet. Allow the edges to set for a minute.
5. Sprinkle crumbled goat cheese evenly over the top of the frittata.
6. Transfer the skillet to the preheated oven and bake for about 15 minutes or until the frittata is set in the middle.
7. Once cooked, remove from the oven and let it cool for a few minutes.

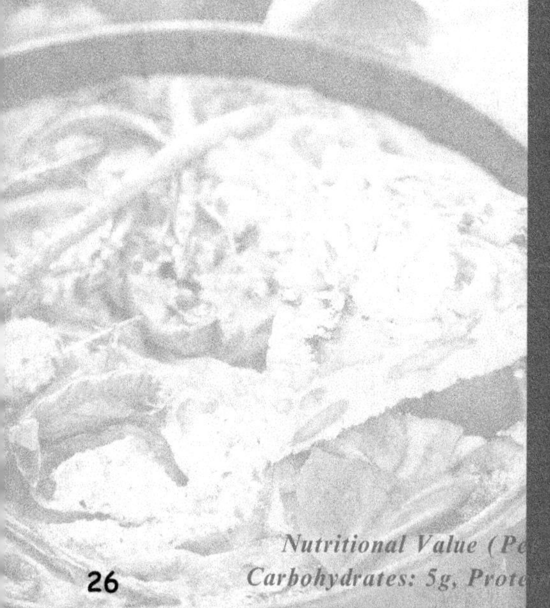

Nutritional Value (Per Serving): Calories: [illegible]
Carbohydrates: 5g, Prote[illegible]

Mediterranean Stuffed Bell Peppers with Ground Turkey

SERVINGS : 2　　**PREP TIME** : 15 MIN　　**COOKING TIME : 30 MIN**

RATINGS :  ★★★★★

INGREDIENTS

- 2 large bell peppers (any color)
- 200g lean ground turkey
- 1/2 cup cooked quinoa
- 1/2 cup diced tomatoes
- 1/4 cup diced red onion
- 2 cloves garlic, minced
- 2 tbsps. chopped fresh parsley
- 1 tbsp. olive oil
- 1 tsp dried oregano
- 1 tsp ground cumin
- Salt and pepper to taste

METHOD

1. Preheat the oven to 375°F (190°C).
2. Cut the tops off the bell peppers and remove seeds and membranes.
3. In a skillet over medium heat, sauté the ground turkey in olive oil until browned. Add garlic, red onion, and cook until softened.
4. In a mixing bowl, combine the cooked quinoa, diced tomatoes, cooked turkey mixture, parsley, oregano, cumin, salt, and pepper.
5. Stuff each bell pepper with the mixture, pressing down gently to pack it.
6. Place stuffed peppers in a baking dish and bake for 25-30 minutes, or until peppers are tender.
7. Serve hot, garnished with additional parsley if desired.

Salmon and Avocado Nori Rolls

SERVINGS : 2   **PREP TIME** : 20 MIN   **COOKING TIME : 10 MIN**

RATINGS : ★★★★★

INGREDIENTS

- 2 sheets nori seaweed
- 200g fresh salmon fillet, thinly sliced
- 1 ripe avocado, sliced
- 1/2 cucumber, julienned
- 1 cup shredded cabbage
- 2 tablespoons sesame seeds
- 2 tablespoons low-sodium soy sauce
- 1 tablespoon rice vinegar
- 1 teaspoon grated ginger
- 1 teaspoon wasabi (optional)
- Salt and pepper to taste

METHOD

1. Lay a sheet of nori on a bamboo sushi rolling mat.
2. Evenly distribute the shredded cabbage on the nori, leaving a small border at the top.
3. Place slices of salmon, avocado, and julienned cucumber on top of the cabbage.
4. Sprinkle sesame seeds evenly over the ingredients.
5. In a small bowl, mix soy sauce, rice vinegar, grated ginger, and wasabi (if using). Drizzle the mixture over the ingredients.
6. Season with salt and pepper to taste.
7. Carefully roll the nori, using the bamboo mat to help create a tight roll. Seal the edge with a dab of water.
8. Repeat the process with the second sheet of nori.
9. Using a sharp knife, slice each roll into bite-sized pieces.
10. Serve with additional soy sauce for dipping.

Nutritional Value (per serving): Calories: 350,
Carbohydrates: 15g, Proteins: 20g, Fats: 20g, Sugar: 2g

Cucumber and Smoked Salmon Bites

SERVINGS : 2   **PREP TIME** : 10 MIN   **COOKING TIME : 0 MIN**

RATINGS : ★★★★★

INGREDIENTS

- 1 medium cucumber, thinly sliced (about 200g or 1 cup)
- 100g smoked salmon, cut into bite-sized pieces
- 2 tbsps. Greek yogurt
- 1 tbsp. fresh dill, chopped
- 1 tsp capers, drained
- 1 tsp lemon juice
- Salt and pepper to taste

METHOD

1. Arrange the cucumber slices on a serving platter.
2. In a small bowl, mix Greek yogurt, fresh dill, capers, and lemon juice.
3. Spoon a small amount of the yogurt mixture onto each cucumber slice.
4. Top each cucumber slice with a piece of smoked salmon.
5. Season with salt and pepper to taste.
6. Serve immediately and enjoy your healthy and delicious snack!

Nutritional Value (Per Serving): Calories: 120, Carbohydrates: 5g, Proteins: 15g, Fats: 5g, Sugar: 2g

Smoked Salmon and Avocado Cups

SERVINGS : 2 **PREP TIME : 10 MIN** **COOKING TIME : 0 MIN**

RATINGS :  ★★★★★

INGREDIENTS

- 150g smoked salmon slices
- 1 large avocado, diced
- 1 cup cucumber, diced
- 1/4 cup red onion, finely chopped
- 2 tablespoons capers
- 1 tablespoon fresh dill, chopped
- 1 tablespoon lemon juice
- Salt and pepper to taste

METHOD

1. In a bowl, combine diced avocado, cucumber, red onion, capers, and fresh dill.
2. Gently fold in smoked salmon slices, ensuring an even distribution of ingredients.
3. Drizzle lemon juice over the mixture and season with salt and pepper to taste. Mix gently.
4. Spoon the smoked salmon and avocado mixture into individual cups or small bowls.
5. Garnish with additional dill if desired.

Nutritional Value (Per Serving): Calories: 250, Carbohydrates: 10g, Proteins: 15g, Fats: 18g, Sugar: 2g

Walnut and Rosemary Roasted Grapes

🍴 **SERVINGS : 2**   🕐 **PREP TIME** : 10 MIN   🕐 **COOKING TIME : 15 MIN**

RATINGS : 

INGREDIENTS

- 2 cups red seedless grapes (about 400g)
- 1/4 cup walnuts, chopped (30g)
- 1 tablespoon fresh rosemary, finely chopped
- 1 tablespoon olive oil (15ml)
- 1/4 teaspoon sea salt
- 1/4 teaspoon black pepper

METHOD

1. Preheat the oven to 375°F (190°C).
2. Rinse and pat dry the grapes. Remove them from the stems and place in a mixing bowl.
3. Toss the grapes with chopped walnuts, finely chopped rosemary, olive oil, sea salt, and black pepper. Ensure the grapes are evenly coated.
4. Spread the grape mixture on a baking sheet lined with parchment paper. Roast in the preheated oven for about 15 minutes or until the grapes start to wrinkle and the walnuts are toasted.
5. Remove from the oven and let it cool slightly. Serve the Walnut and Rosemary Roasted Grapes warm.

Smoky Turmeric Popcorn

SERVINGS : 2   **PREP TIME : 5 MIN**   **COOKING TIME : 10 MIN**

RATINGS : 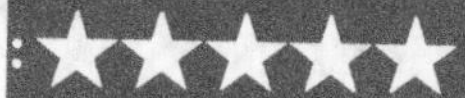

INGREDIENTS

- 1/2 cup popcorn kernels (120g)
- 1 tablespoon olive oil (15ml)
- 1 teaspoon ground turmeric (5g)
- 1/2 teaspoon smoked paprika (2.5g)
- 1/4 teaspoon garlic powder (1.25g)
- 1/4 teaspoon onion powder (1.25g)
- 1/4 teaspoon sea salt (1.5g)

METHOD

1. In a large pot, heat the olive oil over medium heat.
2. Add the popcorn kernels and cover with a lid. Shake the pot occasionally to ensure even popping.
3. Once the popping slows down, remove from heat and let it sit for a minute to ensure any remaining kernels pop.
4. In a small bowl, mix the ground turmeric, smoked paprika, garlic powder, onion powder, and sea salt.
5. Drizzle the spice mixture over the popcorn and toss gently to coat evenly.

Nutritional Value (p
Carbohydrates: 18g, Pro

Almond and Matcha Energy Bites

SERVINGS : 2   **PREP TIME** : 15 MIN   **COOKING TIME : 10 MIN**

RATINGS : ★★★★★

INGREDIENTS

- 1 cup (150g) Almonds, finely ground
- 2 tablespoons (30g) Matcha powder
- 2 tablespoons (30g) Flaxseed meal
- 1/4 cup (60ml) Almond Butter (unsweetened)
- 1/4 cup (60ml) Coconut Milk (unsweetened)
- 1 teaspoon (5g) Vanilla Extract
- A pinch of Salt

METHOD

1. In a mixing bowl, combine finely ground almonds, matcha powder, and flaxseed meal.
2. Add almond butter, coconut milk, vanilla extract, and a pinch of salt to the dry ingredients. Mix well until a dough-like consistency forms.
3. Take small portions of the mixture and roll them into bite-sized balls. Place them on a tray lined with parchment paper.
4. Refrigerate the energy bites for at least 1 hour to help them set.
5. Once chilled, serve and enjoy these healthy Almond and Matcha Energy Bites.

Nutritional Value (Per Serving : Calories 200,
Carbohydrates: 10g, Proteins: 5, Fats 15g. Fiber: 2g

DAILY MEAL PLANNER

DAY/DATE: _______________________________

BREAKFAST

GROCERY LIST

LUNCH

DINNER

SNACKS

NOTES

____

____

____

Beetroot and Dark Chocolate Truffles

SERVINGS : 2   **PREP TIME : 15 MIN**   **COOKING TIME : 0 MIN**

RATINGS : ★★★★★

INGREDIENTS

- 150g beetroot, cooked and finely grated
- 30g unsweetened dark chocolate (at least 70% cocoa), finely chopped
- 2 tbsps. unsweetened cocoa powder
- 1 tbsp. chia seeds
- 1 tbsp. almond flour
- 1/2 tsp vanilla extract
- A pinch of salt

METHOD

1. In a bowl, combine the grated beetroot, chopped dark chocolate, chia seeds, almond flour, vanilla extract, and a pinch of salt.
2. Mix the ingredients thoroughly until well combined.
3. Shape the mixture into small truffle-sized balls using your hands.
4. Roll each truffle in unsweetened cocoa powder until evenly coated.
5. Place the truffles on a plate and refrigerate for at least 1 hour to allow them to firm up.
6. Once chilled, your Beetroot and Dark Chocolate Truffles are ready to be enjoyed!

Nutritional Value (per serving): Calories: approx.
Carbohydrates: 15g, Pro...

Mango Basil Popsicles

RATINGS : ★★★★★

INGREDIENTS

- 2 cups fresh ripe mango, peeled and diced (about 400g)
- 1/4 cup fresh basil leaves, finely chopped
- 1/2 cup Greek yogurt (unsweetened)
- 1/2 teaspoon lime zest
- 1 tablespoon lime juice
- 1/2 cup water

METHOD

1. In a blender, combine diced mango, chopped basil, Greek yogurt, lime zest, lime juice, and water.
2. Blend until smooth and well combined.
3. Pour the mixture into Popsicle molds, leaving a little space at the top for expansion.
4. Insert Popsicle sticks into the molds.
5. Freeze for at least 4 hours or until completely set.
6. Once frozen, run the molds under warm water to release the popsicles easily.

Nutritional Value (Per Serving): Calories: 110 kcal, Carbohydrates: 21g, Proteins: 5g, Fats: 1g, Sugar: 15g

Spiced Carrot and Coconut Bites

SERVINGS : 2 **PREP TIME** : 15 MIN **COOKING TIME : 0 MIN**

RATINGS : 

INGREDIENTS

- 200g (about 1 1/2 cups) grated carrots
- 50g (1/2 cup) unsweetened shredded coconut
- 30g (1/4 cup) almond flour
- 1 tsp ground cinnamon
- 1/2 tsp ground nutmeg
- 1/4 tsp ground ginger
- 1/4 tsp ground cloves
- 1/4 cup unsweetened applesauce
- 1/4 cup chopped walnuts
- 1/4 cup ground flaxseed
- A pinch of salt

METHOD

1. In a large mixing bowl, combine grated carrots, shredded coconut, almond flour, ground cinnamon, ground nutmeg, ground ginger, ground cloves, applesauce, chopped walnuts, ground flaxseed, and a pinch of salt.
2. Mix the ingredients thoroughly until well combined. The applesauce will help bind the mixture.
3. Using your hands, form the mixture into bite-sized balls. If the mixture is too sticky, you can wet your hands slightly.
4. Place the carrot and coconut bites on a plate or tray and refrigerate for at least 1 hour to firm up.
5. Once chilled, the bites are ready to be enjoyed.

Chickpea Flour Banana Bread

RATINGS :  ★★★★★

INGREDIENTS

- 1 large ripe banana, mashed (about 200g or 1 cup)
- 1 cup chickpea flour (120g)
- 1/2 teaspoon baking soda
- 1/2 teaspoon cinnamon
- 1/4 teaspoon nutmeg
- 1/4 teaspoon salt
- 1 egg
- 1/4 cup unsweetened almond milk (60ml)
- 1 teaspoon vanilla extract
- 1/4 cup chopped walnuts (30g)

METHOD

1. Preheat the oven to 350°F (175°C). Grease a small loaf pan.
2. In a large bowl, combine chickpea flour, baking soda, cinnamon, nutmeg, and salt.
3. In a separate bowl, mix mashed banana, egg, almond milk, and vanilla extract.
4. Add the wet ingredients to the dry ingredients and stir until just combined. Fold in chopped walnuts.
5. Pour the batter into the prepared loaf pan.
6. Bake for 25 minutes or until a toothpick inserted into the center comes out clean.
7. Allow the banana bread to cool in the pan for 10 minutes before transferring it to a wire rack to cool completely.

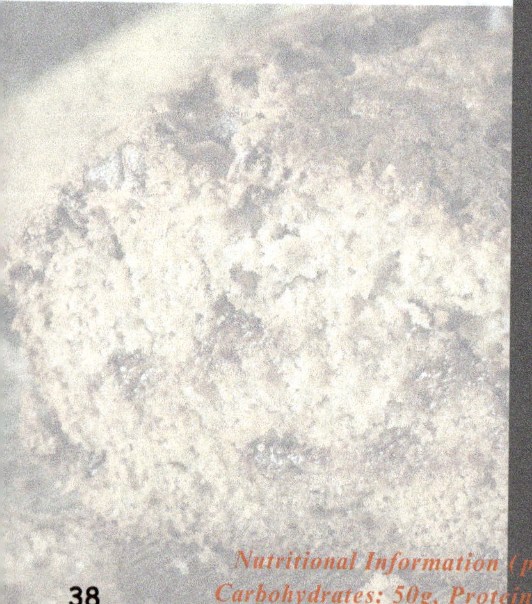

Nutritional Information (per serving): Calories: 350, Carbohydrates: 50g, Proteins: 14g, Fats: 12g, Sugar: 12g

Avocado Lime Mousse

🍴 SERVINGS : 2   🕐 PREP TIME : 10 MIN   🕐 COOKING TIME : 0 MIN

RATINGS  : ★★★★★

INGREDIENTS

- 2 ripe avocados (about 400g), peeled and pitted
- 1/4 cup (60ml) lime juice
- Zest of 1 lime
- 1/4 cup (60ml) unsweetened almond milk
- 2 tablespoons (30ml) Greek yogurt
- 1 teaspoon (5ml) vanilla extract
- Stevia or erythritol, to taste (optional)
- Fresh mint leaves for garnish (optional)

METHOD

1. In a blender or food processor, combine ripe avocados, lime juice, lime zest, almond milk, Greek yogurt, and vanilla extract.
2. Blend the mixture until smooth and creamy. If a sweeter taste is desired, add stevia or erythritol to taste, blending again to combine.
3. Taste and adjust the lime juice or sweetener if necessary to achieve the desired balance.
4. Divide the mousse into two serving glasses or bowls.
5. Refrigerate for at least 30 minutes to allow the mousse to chill and flavors to meld.
6. Garnish with fresh mint leaves before serving, if desired.

DAILY MEAL PLANNER

DAY/DATE: _______________________

BREAKFAST

GROCERY LIST

LUNCH

DINNER

SNACKS

NOTES

Cucumber Mint Delight

SERVINGS : 2   **PREP TIME : 10 MIN**   **COOKING TIME : 0 MIN**

RATINGS : 

INGREDIENTS

- 1 medium cucumber, peeled and chopped (about 200g or 1 cup)
- 1 cup plain Greek yogurt (240ml)
- 1 cup fresh spinach leaves (30g)
- 1/2 cup fresh mint leaves, loosely packed (15g)
- 1/2 avocado, peeled and pitted (about 100g)
- 1 cup ice cubes (240ml)
- 1 tablespoon chia seeds (15g)
- 1 tablespoon flaxseeds (15g)
- 1 cup water (240ml)
- Juice of 1 lime

METHOD

1. Place cucumber, Greek yogurt, spinach, mint, avocado, ice cubes, chia seeds, flaxseeds, water, and lime juice in a blender.
2. Blend until smooth and creamy.
3. Pour into glasses and garnish with a mint leaf if desired.

Nutritional Value (Pe...
Carbohydrates: 10g, Pro...

Spicy Green Apple Smoothie

SERVINGS : 2 **PREP TIME : 10 MIN** **COOKING TIME : 0 MIN**

RATINGS : 

INGREDIENTS

- 2 medium green apples, cored and chopped (about 300g or 2 cups)
- 1 cup cucumber, peeled and diced (about 150g)
- 1 cup spinach leaves, packed (about 30g)
- 1/2 small avocado, peeled and pitted (about 75g)
- 1/2 teaspoon fresh ginger, grated
- 1/4 teaspoon cayenne pepper (adjust to taste)
- 1 cup unsweetened almond milk (240ml)
- 1 cup ice cubes (optional)
- Fresh mint leaves for garnish (optional)

METHOD

1. In a blender, combine chopped green apples, diced cucumber, spinach leaves, avocado, grated ginger, and cayenne pepper.
2. Pour in unsweetened almond milk.
3. Blend on high speed until the mixture is smooth and creamy. Add ice cubes if a colder consistency is desired.
4. Taste and adjust the spiciness by adding more cayenne pepper if needed.
5. Pour into glasses, garnish with fresh mint leaves if desired, and serve immediately.

Nutritional Value (Per Serving): Calories: 120, Carbohydrates: 20g, Proteins: 3g, Fats: 5g, Sugars: 10g.

Turmeric Pineapple Fusion

🍴 **SERVINGS : 2**   🕐 **PREP TIME** : 10 MIN   🕐 **COOKING TIME : 0 MIN**

RATINGS : 

INGREDIENTS

- 1 cup (240 ml) unsweetened almond milk
- 1 cup (150 g) fresh pineapple chunks
- 1 medium cucumber, peeled and sliced
- 1 small banana, peeled
- 1 teaspoon turmeric powder
- 1/2 teaspoon ground ginger
- 1/2 teaspoon cinnamon
- 1 scoop (about 30 g) plant-based protein powder
- Ice cubes (optional)

METHOD

1. In a blender, combine almond milk, pineapple chunks, cucumber slices, banana, turmeric powder, ground ginger, cinnamon, and plant-based protein powder.
2. Blend until smooth and creamy. If a thicker consistency is desired, add ice cubes and blend again.
3. Pour the smoothie into two glasses and serve immediately.

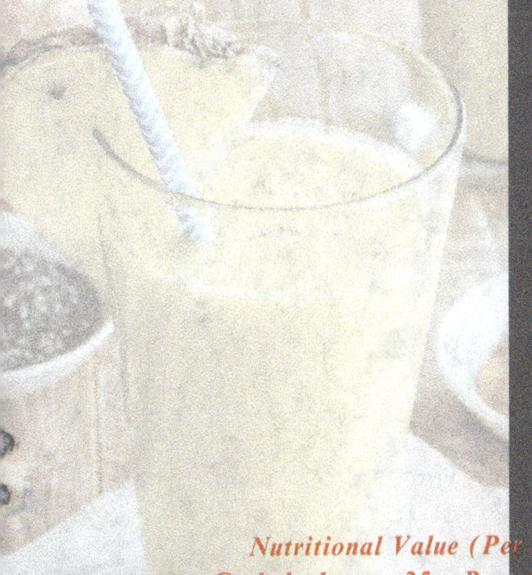

Nutritional Value (Per Serving): Calories: 120, Carbohydrates: 25g, Proteins: 8g, Fats: 2g, Sugar: 12g

Carrot Ginger Elixir

SERVINGS : 2 **PREP TIME : 10 MIN** **COOKING TIME : 0 MIN**

RATINGS : 

INGREDIENTS

- 2 medium-sized carrots, peeled and chopped (about 200g or 1 cup)
- 1-inch piece of fresh ginger, peeled and grated (about 12g)
- 1 cup cucumber, peeled and diced (about 150g)
- 1 cup unsweetened almond milk (240ml)
- 1/2 cup Greek yogurt, plain, non-fat (120g)
- 1 tablespoon chia seeds (15g)
- Ice cubes (optional)

METHOD

1. In a blender, combine chopped carrots, grated ginger, diced cucumber, almond milk, Greek yogurt, and chia seeds.
2. Blend until smooth. If the smoothie is too thick, you can add a bit more almond milk to reach your desired consistency.
3. Add ice cubes if a colder temperature is preferred and blend again until well mixed.
4. Pour the smoothie into glasses and enjoy immediately.

Nutritional Value (per serving): Calories: 110, Carbohydrates: 15g, Protein: 6g, Fat: 3g, Sugar: 7g,

Dear Readers,

Congratulations on reaching the end of "Prediabetes Recipes"! I extend my heartfelt thanks to each of you for embarking on this culinary journey towards healthier living.

I sincerely hope you enjoyed experimenting with the 30 thoughtfully crafted recipes designed to support a prediabetic lifestyle. Your commitment to exploring these delicious and nutritious options is commendable.

In summary, "Prediabetes Recipes" is a collection born out of my passion for making balanced and flavorful choices, catering specifically to those on the prediabetes spectrum. Each recipe has been carefully curated to not only tantalize your taste buds but also contribute to better blood sugar management.

As you continue on your health-conscious path, here are a few pieces of advice:
Mindful Eating: Pay attention to portion sizes and savor each bite mindfully.
Regular Exercise: Incorporate regular physical activity into your routine to enhance overall well-being.
Hydration is Key: Drink plenty of water throughout the day to stay hydrated.
Avoiding processed sugars and refined carbohydrates will be beneficial for your journey ahead. Remember, small changes can lead to significant health improvements.

I genuinely appreciate your support as an independent publisher, and your feedback means the world to me. If you enjoyed the recipes or have suggestions, I'd love to hear from you. Reach out to me at eatwithpeggymorgan@gmail.com. Pretty please, leave your reviews on Amazon; they are invaluable and will guide me in crafting future culinary adventures. Your reviews on Amazon will not only help others discover the book but will also provide insights into the impact of these recipes on your health journey.

Don't forget to explore my other books, and keep an eye out for upcoming releases. Thank you once again for choosing "Prediabetes Recipes." Wishing you a vibrant and health-filled future!

Warm regards,

Peggy R. Morgan
Author, "Prediabetes Recipes"

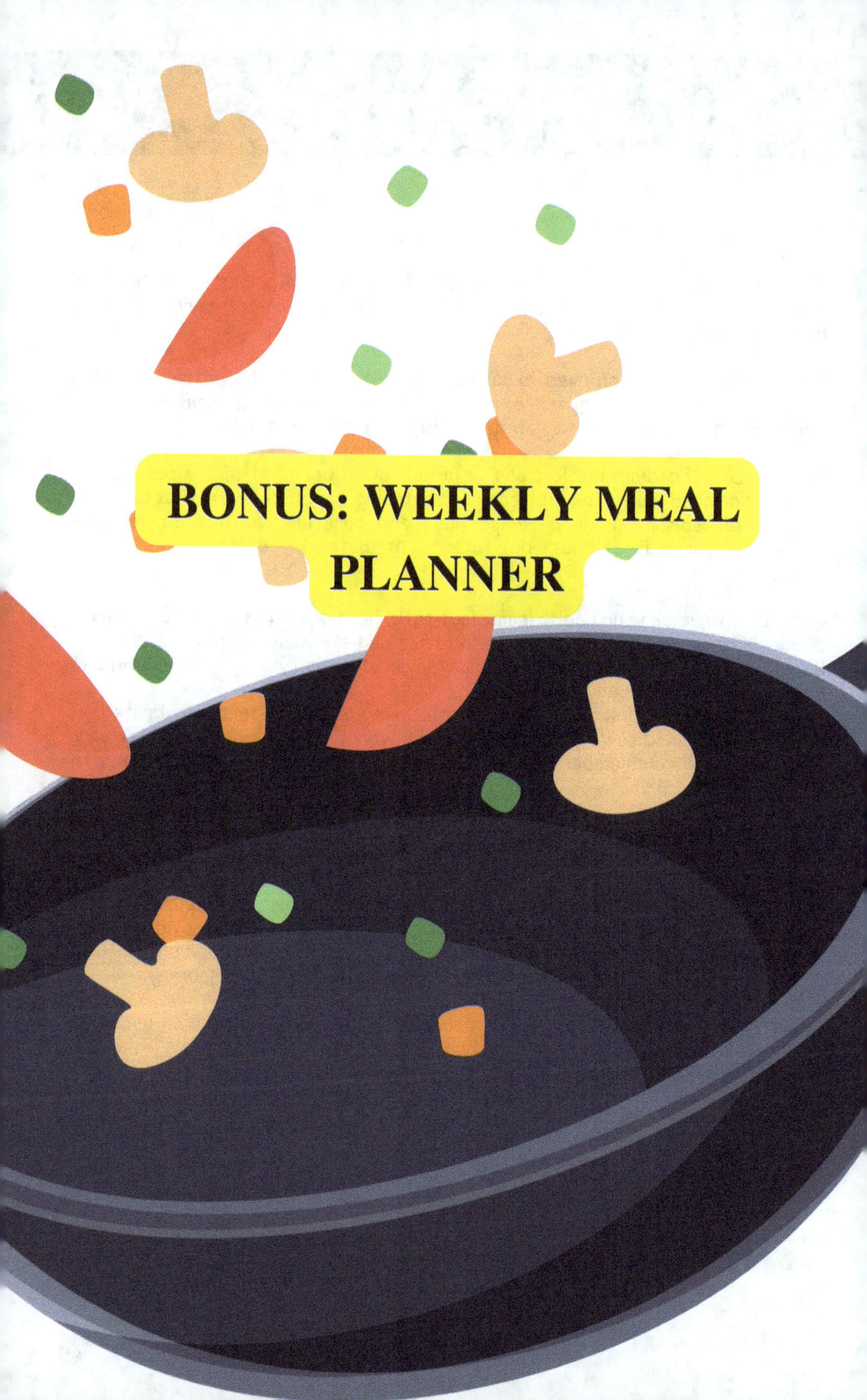

BONUS: WEEKLY MEAL PLANNER

WEEKLY MEAL PLANNER

MONDAY	BREAKFAST	
	LUNCH	
	DINNER	
TUESDAY	BREAKFAST	
	LUNCH	
	DINNER	
WEDNESDAY	BREAKFAST	
	LUNCH	
	DINNER	
THURSDAY	BREAKFAST	
	LUNCH	
	DINNER	
FRIDAY	BREAKFAST	
	LUNCH	
	DINNER	
SATURDAY	BREAKFAST	
	LUNCH	
	DINNER	
SUNDAY	BREAKFAST	
	LUNCH	
	DINNER	

GROCERY LIST

SNACKS

WEEKLY MEAL PLANNER

MONDAY	BREAKFAST	
	LUNCH	
	DINNER	

TUESDAY	BREAKFAST	
	LUNCH	
	DINNER	

WEDNESDAY	BREAKFAST	
	LUNCH	
	DINNER	

THURSDAY	BREAKFAST	
	LUNCH	
	DINNER	

FRIDAY	BREAKFAST	
	LUNCH	
	DINNER	

SATURDAY	BREAKFAST	
	LUNCH	
	DINNER	

SUNDAY	BREAKFAST	
	LUNCH	
	DINNER	

GROCERY LIST

SNACKS

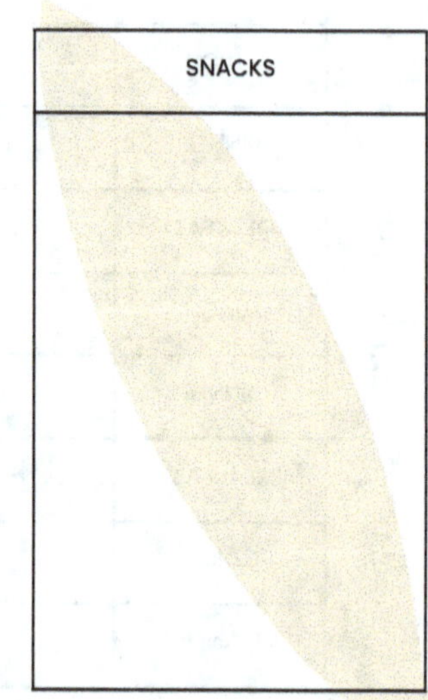

WEEKLY MEAL PLANNER

MONDAY	BREAKFAST	
	LUNCH	
	DINNER	
TUESDAY	BREAKFAST	
	LUNCH	
	DINNER	
WEDNESDAY	BREAKFAST	
	LUNCH	
	DINNER	
THURSDAY	BREAKFAST	
	LUNCH	
	DINNER	
FRIDAY	BREAKFAST	
	LUNCH	
	DINNER	
SATURDAY	BREAKFAST	
	LUNCH	
	DINNER	
SUNDAY	BREAKFAST	
	LUNCH	
	DINNER	

GROCERY LIST

SNACKS

WEEKLY MEAL PLANNER

MONDAY	BREAKFAST	
	LUNCH	
	DINNER	

TUESDAY	BREAKFAST	
	LUNCH	
	DINNER	

WEDNESDAY	BREAKFAST	
	LUNCH	
	DINNER	

THURSDAY	BREAKFAST	
	LUNCH	
	DINNER	

FRIDAY	BREAKFAST	
	LUNCH	
	DINNER	

SATURDAY	BREAKFAST	
	LUNCH	
	DINNER	

SUNDAY	BREAKFAST	
	LUNCH	
	DINNER	

GROCERY LIST

SNACKS

WEEKLY MEAL PLANNER

MONDAY	BREAKFAST	
	LUNCH	
	DINNER	
TUESDAY	BREAKFAST	
	LUNCH	
	DINNER	
WEDNESDAY	BREAKFAST	
	LUNCH	
	DINNER	
THURSDAY	BREAKFAST	
	LUNCH	
	DINNER	
FRIDAY	BREAKFAST	
	LUNCH	
	DINNER	
SATURDAY	BREAKFAST	
	LUNCH	
	DINNER	
SUNDAY	BREAKFAST	
	LUNCH	
	DINNER	

GROCERY LIST

SNACKS

WEEKLY MEAL PLANNER

MONDAY		
	BREAKFAST	
	LUNCH	
	DINNER	

TUESDAY		
	BREAKFAST	
	LUNCH	
	DINNER	

WEDNESDAY		
	BREAKFAST	
	LUNCH	
	DINNER	

THURSDAY		
	BREAKFAST	
	LUNCH	
	DINNER	

FRIDAY		
	BREAKFAST	
	LUNCH	
	DINNER	

SATURDAY		
	BREAKFAST	
	LUNCH	
	DINNER	

SUNDAY		
	BREAKFAST	
	LUNCH	
	DINNER	

GROCERY LIST

SNACKS

WEEKLY MEAL PLANNER

MONDAY	BREAKFAST	
	LUNCH	
	DINNER	
TUESDAY	BREAKFAST	
	LUNCH	
	DINNER	
WEDNESDAY	BREAKFAST	
	LUNCH	
	DINNER	
THURSDAY	BREAKFAST	
	LUNCH	
	DINNER	
FRIDAY	BREAKFAST	
	LUNCH	
	DINNER	
SATURDAY	BREAKFAST	
	LUNCH	
	DINNER	
SUNDAY	BREAKFAST	
	LUNCH	
	DINNER	

GROCERY LIST

SNACKS

WEEKLY MEAL PLANNER

MONDAY	BREAKFAST	
	LUNCH	
	DINNER	
TUESDAY	BREAKFAST	
	LUNCH	
	DINNER	
WEDNESDAY	BREAKFAST	
	LUNCH	
	DINNER	
THURSDAY	BREAKFAST	
	LUNCH	
	DINNER	
FRIDAY	BREAKFAST	
	LUNCH	
	DINNER	
SATURDAY	BREAKFAST	
	LUNCH	
	DINNER	
SUNDAY	BREAKFAST	
	LUNCH	
	DINNER	

GROCERY LIST

SNACKS

WEEKLY MEAL PLANNER

MONDAY	BREAKFAST	
	LUNCH	
	DINNER	

TUESDAY	BREAKFAST	
	LUNCH	
	DINNER	

WEDNESDAY	BREAKFAST	
	LUNCH	
	DINNER	

THURSDAY	BREAKFAST	
	LUNCH	
	DINNER	

FRIDAY	BREAKFAST	
	LUNCH	
	DINNER	

SATURDAY	BREAKFAST	
	LUNCH	
	DINNER	

SUNDAY	BREAKFAST	
	LUNCH	
	DINNER	

GROCERY LIST

SNACKS

WEEKLY MEAL PLANNER

MONDAY	BREAKFAST	
	LUNCH	
	DINNER	
TUESDAY	BREAKFAST	
	LUNCH	
	DINNER	
WEDNESDAY	BREAKFAST	
	LUNCH	
	DINNER	
THURSDAY	BREAKFAST	
	LUNCH	
	DINNER	
FRIDAY	BREAKFAST	
	LUNCH	
	DINNER	
SATURDAY	BREAKFAST	
	LUNCH	
	DINNER	
SUNDAY	BREAKFAST	
	LUNCH	
	DINNER	

GROCERY LIST

SNACKS

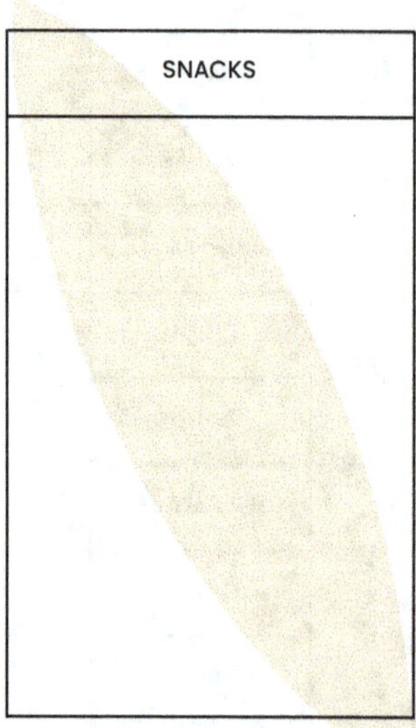

WEEKLY MEAL PLANNER

MONDAY	BREAKFAST	
	LUNCH	
	DINNER	

TUESDAY	BREAKFAST	
	LUNCH	
	DINNER	

WEDNESDAY	BREAKFAST	
	LUNCH	
	DINNER	

THURSDAY	BREAKFAST	
	LUNCH	
	DINNER	

FRIDAY	BREAKFAST	
	LUNCH	
	DINNER	

SATURDAY	BREAKFAST	
	LUNCH	
	DINNER	

SUNDAY	BREAKFAST	
	LUNCH	
	DINNER	

GROCERY LIST

SNACKS

WEEKLY MEAL PLANNER

MONDAY	BREAKFAST	
	LUNCH	
	DINNER	
TUESDAY	BREAKFAST	
	LUNCH	
	DINNER	
WEDNESDAY	BREAKFAST	
	LUNCH	
	DINNER	
THURSDAY	BREAKFAST	
	LUNCH	
	DINNER	
FRIDAY	BREAKFAST	
	LUNCH	
	DINNER	
SATURDAY	BREAKFAST	
	LUNCH	
	DINNER	
SUNDAY	BREAKFAST	
	LUNCH	
	DINNER	

GROCERY LIST

SNACKS

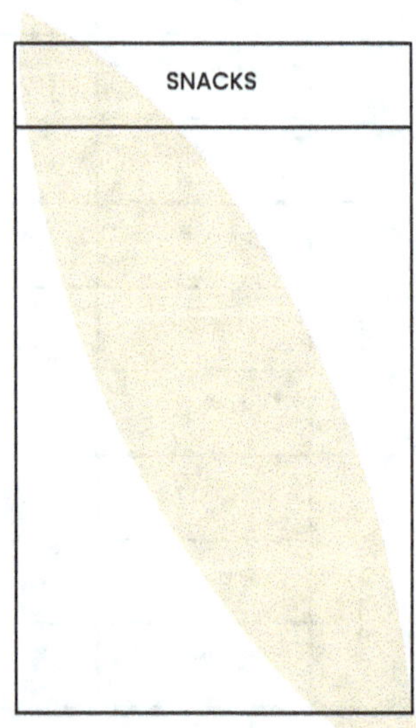

WEEKLY MEAL PLANNER

MONDAY		
	BREAKFAST	
	LUNCH	
	DINNER	

TUESDAY		
	BREAKFAST	
	LUNCH	
	DINNER	

WEDNESDAY		
	BREAKFAST	
	LUNCH	
	DINNER	

THURSDAY		
	BREAKFAST	
	LUNCH	
	DINNER	

FRIDAY		
	BREAKFAST	
	LUNCH	
	DINNER	

SATURDAY		
	BREAKFAST	
	LUNCH	
	DINNER	

SUNDAY		
	BREAKFAST	
	LUNCH	
	DINNER	

GROCERY LIST

SNACKS

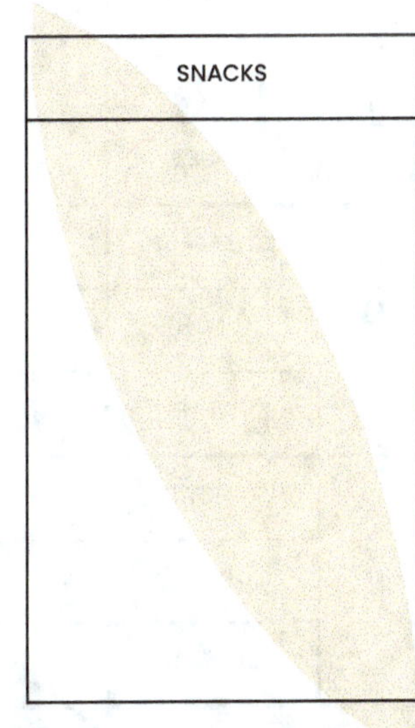

WEEKLY MEAL PLANNER

MONDAY	BREAKFAST	
	LUNCH	
	DINNER	
TUESDAY	BREAKFAST	
	LUNCH	
	DINNER	
WEDNESDAY	BREAKFAST	
	LUNCH	
	DINNER	
THURSDAY	BREAKFAST	
	LUNCH	
	DINNER	
FRIDAY	BREAKFAST	
	LUNCH	
	DINNER	
SATURDAY	BREAKFAST	
	LUNCH	
	DINNER	
SUNDAY	BREAKFAST	
	LUNCH	
	DINNER	

GROCERY LIST

SNACKS

WEEKLY MEAL PLANNER

MONDAY

BREAKFAST	
LUNCH	
DINNER	

TUESDAY

BREAKFAST	
LUNCH	
DINNER	

WEDNESDAY

BREAKFAST	
LUNCH	
DINNER	

THURSDAY

BREAKFAST	
LUNCH	
DINNER	

FRIDAY

BREAKFAST	
LUNCH	
DINNER	

SATURDAY

BREAKFAST	
LUNCH	
DINNER	

SUNDAY

BREAKFAST	
LUNCH	
DINNER	

GROCERY LIST

SNACKS

WEEKLY MEAL PLANNER

MONDAY	BREAKFAST	
	LUNCH	
	DINNER	
TUESDAY	BREAKFAST	
	LUNCH	
	DINNER	
WEDNESDAY	BREAKFAST	
	LUNCH	
	DINNER	
THURSDAY	BREAKFAST	
	LUNCH	
	DINNER	
FRIDAY	BREAKFAST	
	LUNCH	
	DINNER	
SATURDAY	BREAKFAST	
	LUNCH	
	DINNER	
SUNDAY	BREAKFAST	
	LUNCH	
	DINNER	

GROCERY LIST

SNACKS

WEEKLY MEAL PLANNER

MONDAY	BREAKFAST	
	LUNCH	
	DINNER	
TUESDAY	BREAKFAST	
	LUNCH	
	DINNER	
WEDNESDAY	BREAKFAST	
	LUNCH	
	DINNER	
THURSDAY	BREAKFAST	
	LUNCH	
	DINNER	
FRIDAY	BREAKFAST	
	LUNCH	
	DINNER	
SATURDAY	BREAKFAST	
	LUNCH	
	DINNER	
SUNDAY	BREAKFAST	
	LUNCH	
	DINNER	

GROCERY LIST

SNACKS

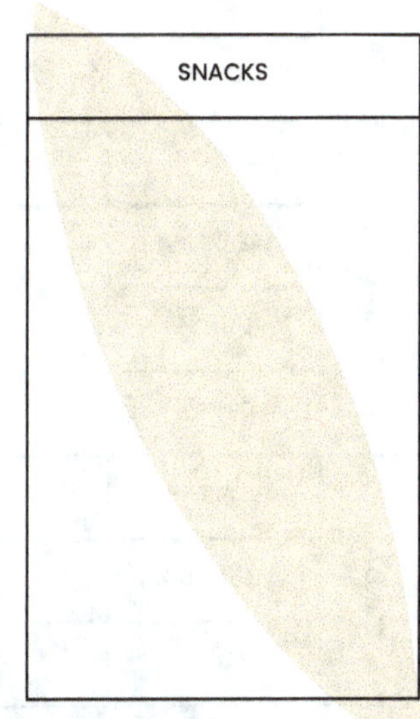

WEEKLY MEAL PLANNER

MONDAY	BREAKFAST	
	LUNCH	
	DINNER	

TUESDAY	BREAKFAST	
	LUNCH	
	DINNER	

WEDNESDAY	BREAKFAST	
	LUNCH	
	DINNER	

THURSDAY	BREAKFAST	
	LUNCH	
	DINNER	

FRIDAY	BREAKFAST	
	LUNCH	
	DINNER	

SATURDAY	BREAKFAST	
	LUNCH	
	DINNER	

SUNDAY	BREAKFAST	
	LUNCH	
	DINNER	

GROCERY LIST

SNACKS

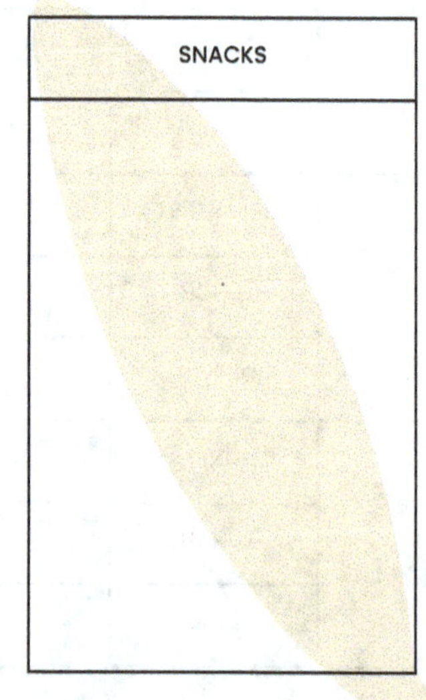

WEEKLY MEAL PLANNER

MONDAY	BREAKFAST	
	LUNCH	
	DINNER	
TUESDAY	BREAKFAST	
	LUNCH	
	DINNER	
WEDNESDAY	BREAKFAST	
	LUNCH	
	DINNER	
THURSDAY	BREAKFAST	
	LUNCH	
	DINNER	
FRIDAY	BREAKFAST	
	LUNCH	
	DINNER	
SATURDAY	BREAKFAST	
	LUNCH	
	DINNER	
SUNDAY	BREAKFAST	
	LUNCH	
	DINNER	

GROCERY LIST

SNACKS

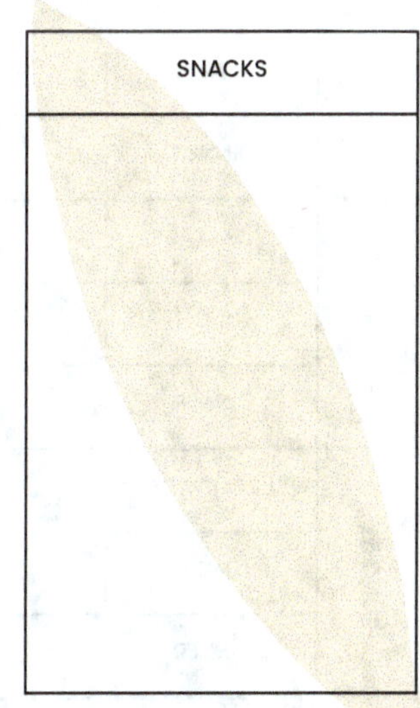

WEEKLY MEAL PLANNER

MONDAY	BREAKFAST	
	LUNCH	
	DINNER	
TUESDAY	BREAKFAST	
	LUNCH	
	DINNER	
WEDNESDAY	BREAKFAST	
	LUNCH	
	DINNER	
THURSDAY	BREAKFAST	
	LUNCH	
	DINNER	
FRIDAY	BREAKFAST	
	LUNCH	
	DINNER	
SATURDAY	BREAKFAST	
	LUNCH	
	DINNER	
SUNDAY	BREAKFAST	
	LUNCH	
	DINNER	

GROCERY LIST

SNACKS

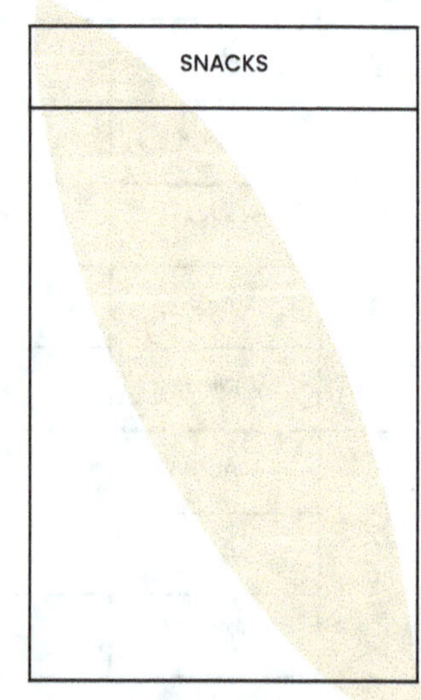

WEEKLY MEAL PLANNER

MONDAY	BREAKFAST	
	LUNCH	
	DINNER	

TUESDAY	BREAKFAST	
	LUNCH	
	DINNER	

WEDNESDAY	BREAKFAST	
	LUNCH	
	DINNER	

THURSDAY	BREAKFAST	
	LUNCH	
	DINNER	

FRIDAY	BREAKFAST	
	LUNCH	
	DINNER	

SATURDAY	BREAKFAST	
	LUNCH	
	DINNER	

SUNDAY	BREAKFAST	
	LUNCH	
	DINNER	

GROCERY LIST

SNACKS

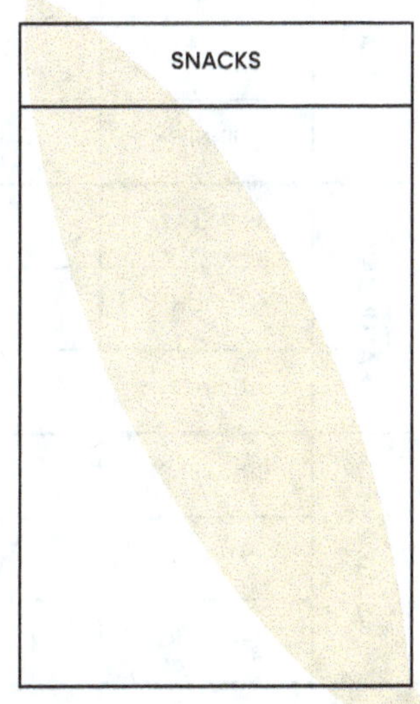

WEEKLY MEAL PLANNER

MONDAY	BREAKFAST	
	LUNCH	
	DINNER	
TUESDAY	BREAKFAST	
	LUNCH	
	DINNER	
WEDNESDAY	BREAKFAST	
	LUNCH	
	DINNER	
THURSDAY	BREAKFAST	
	LUNCH	
	DINNER	
FRIDAY	BREAKFAST	
	LUNCH	
	DINNER	
SATURDAY	BREAKFAST	
	LUNCH	
	DINNER	
SUNDAY	BREAKFAST	
	LUNCH	
	DINNER	

GROCERY LIST

SNACKS

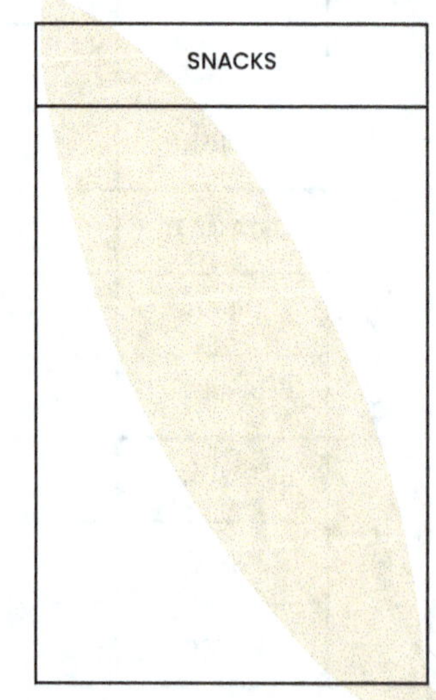

WEEKLY MEAL PLANNER

MONDAY	BREAKFAST	
	LUNCH	
	DINNER	
TUESDAY	BREAKFAST	
	LUNCH	
	DINNER	
WEDNESDAY	BREAKFAST	
	LUNCH	
	DINNER	
THURSDAY	BREAKFAST	
	LUNCH	
	DINNER	
FRIDAY	BREAKFAST	
	LUNCH	
	DINNER	
SATURDAY	BREAKFAST	
	LUNCH	
	DINNER	
SUNDAY	BREAKFAST	
	LUNCH	
	DINNER	

GROCERY LIST

SNACKS

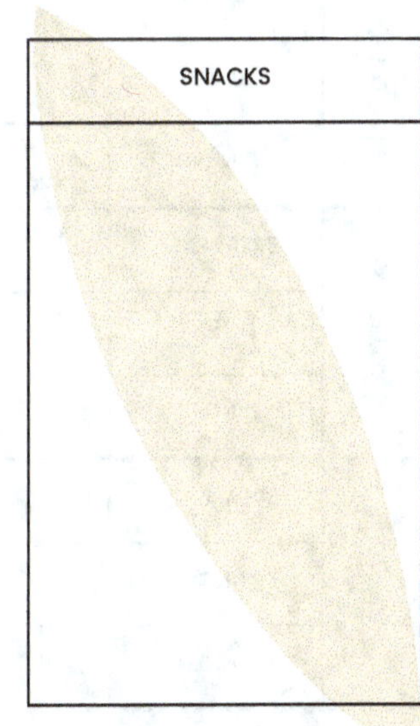

WEEKLY MEAL PLANNER

MONDAY	BREAKFAST	
	LUNCH	
	DINNER	
TUESDAY	BREAKFAST	
	LUNCH	
	DINNER	
WEDNESDAY	BREAKFAST	
	LUNCH	
	DINNER	
THURSDAY	BREAKFAST	
	LUNCH	
	DINNER	
FRIDAY	BREAKFAST	
	LUNCH	
	DINNER	
SATURDAY	BREAKFAST	
	LUNCH	
	DINNER	
SUNDAY	BREAKFAST	
	LUNCH	
	DINNER	

GROCERY LIST

SNACKS

WEEKLY MEAL PLANNER

MONDAY		
	BREAKFAST	
	LUNCH	
	DINNER	

TUESDAY		
	BREAKFAST	
	LUNCH	
	DINNER	

WEDNESDAY		
	BREAKFAST	
	LUNCH	
	DINNER	

THURSDAY		
	BREAKFAST	
	LUNCH	
	DINNER	

FRIDAY		
	BREAKFAST	
	LUNCH	
	DINNER	

SATURDAY		
	BREAKFAST	
	LUNCH	
	DINNER	

SUNDAY		
	BREAKFAST	
	LUNCH	
	DINNER	

GROCERY LIST

SNACKS

WEEKLY MEAL PLANNER

MONDAY

BREAKFAST	
LUNCH	
DINNER	

TUESDAY

BREAKFAST	
LUNCH	
DINNER	

WEDNESDAY

BREAKFAST	
LUNCH	
DINNER	

THURSDAY

BREAKFAST	
LUNCH	
DINNER	

FRIDAY

BREAKFAST	
LUNCH	
DINNER	

SATURDAY

BREAKFAST	
LUNCH	
DINNER	

SUNDAY

BREAKFAST	
LUNCH	
DINNER	

GROCERY LIST

SNACKS

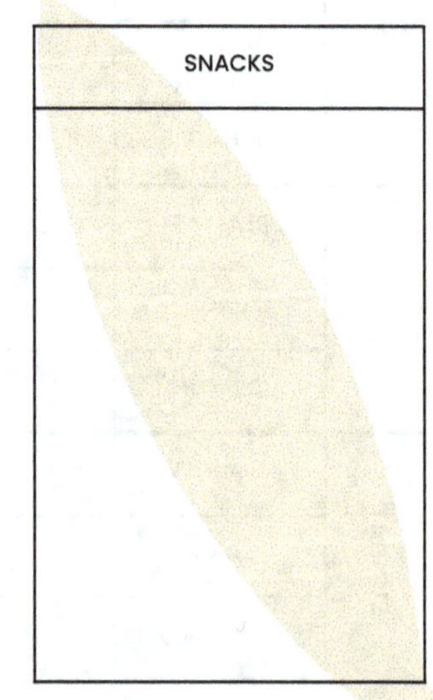